Limited Edition Journal

Published by Dr. Elizabeth Slusher
www.mypricelessdreams.com
© 2021
Illustrations by © FOS, EJE Selects, Mariat, Mujka

For permissions contact:
hello@pricelessdreamsdesigns.com

Dedicated to the Warrior Marquita Moore

Marquita Moore-a wife, mother of three adult children, a new grandmother to her precious grandson; is a two-time breast and colon cancer warrior! In January of 2019 she was diagnosed with Colon and Breast Cancer. She underwent her first double surgery fifteen days after diagnosis. A month later she had another surgery; a lumpectomy. Two months following, she underwent a double mastectomy and reconstructive surgery. She then began chemotherapy treatments and initiatlly rang the bell for finishing chemotherapy on November 15th 2019. In February 2020, the cancer returned and Marquita is actively fighting with a smile on her face, her husband by her side, her children as her strength, her ray of hope grandson in her arms, an encouraging word for anyone , and crafting/creating in her soul and spirit as she continues to claim the victory! Marquita Moore-A Pearl.

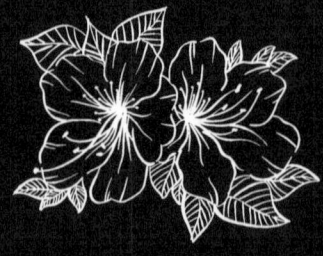

KNOWING YOURSELF
BETTER

Rules here: don't think too hard, just write. A lot of times, the first thing that comes to mind is the right thing.

Q1   **I feel so good when...**

Q2   **What is my support system?**

Q3   **What are my values?**

Q4 What do I like to do for fun?

Q5 What are my short-term goals?

Q6 What am I worried about?

Q7 What's something you love about yourself?

Date:

Self-Care Challenge

Drink More Water	Take A Relaxing Bath	Set Goals For The Next Month
Learn A New Hobby	Find A New Podcast To LIsten to	Write Out A Bucket List
Disconnect From Social Media For One Day	Celebrate A Small Win From The Day	Get 8 Hours Of Sleep
Wear Your Favorite Comfy Outfit All day	Do 30 Minutes Of Yoga	Read A Book

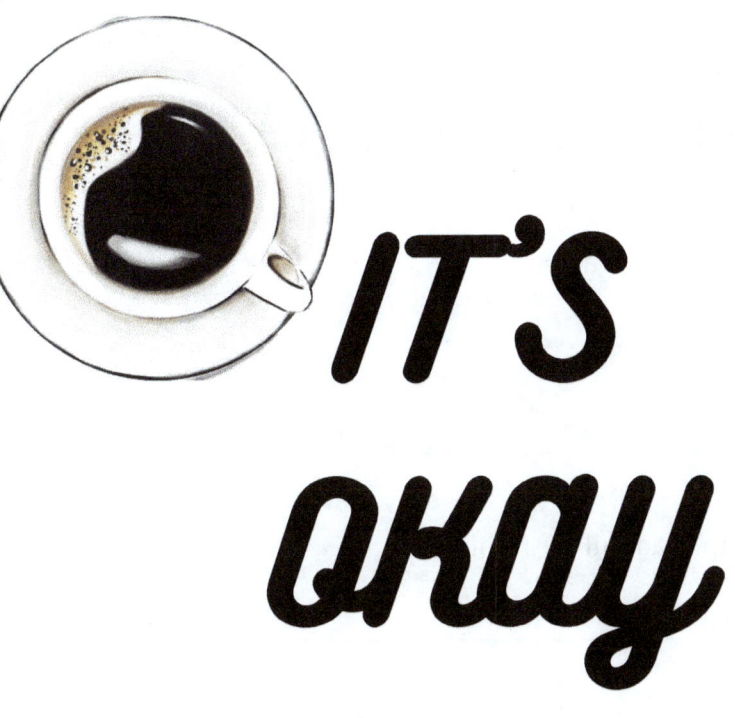

IT'S
okay

★ To make mistake

★ To have bad days

★ To be less than perfect

★ To do what's best for you

★ To Be Yourself

Self-Care Q&A

How do I feel today?

_____

What I am thankful for right now?

_____

What negative attitude do I need to change?

_____

What positive affirmation was I able to
give myself today?

_____

What ongoing support do I need?

_____

What do I need to do to be a better version of myself?

_____

LIFE iS TOUGH BUT SO Are You

Date:

THE BEST VIEW COMES AFTER THE HARDEST CLIMB

Date:

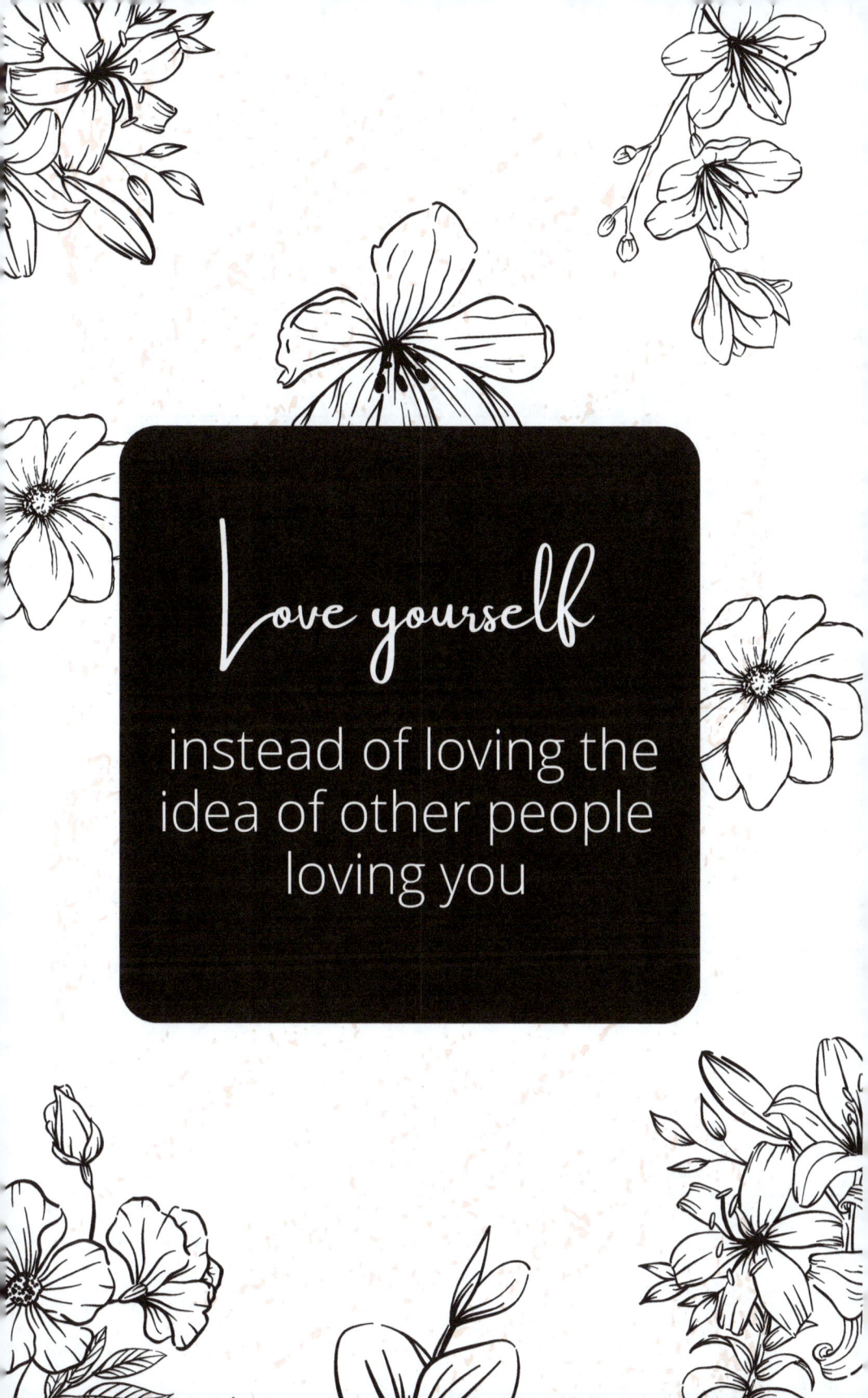

Love yourself

instead of loving the
idea of other people
loving you

Date:

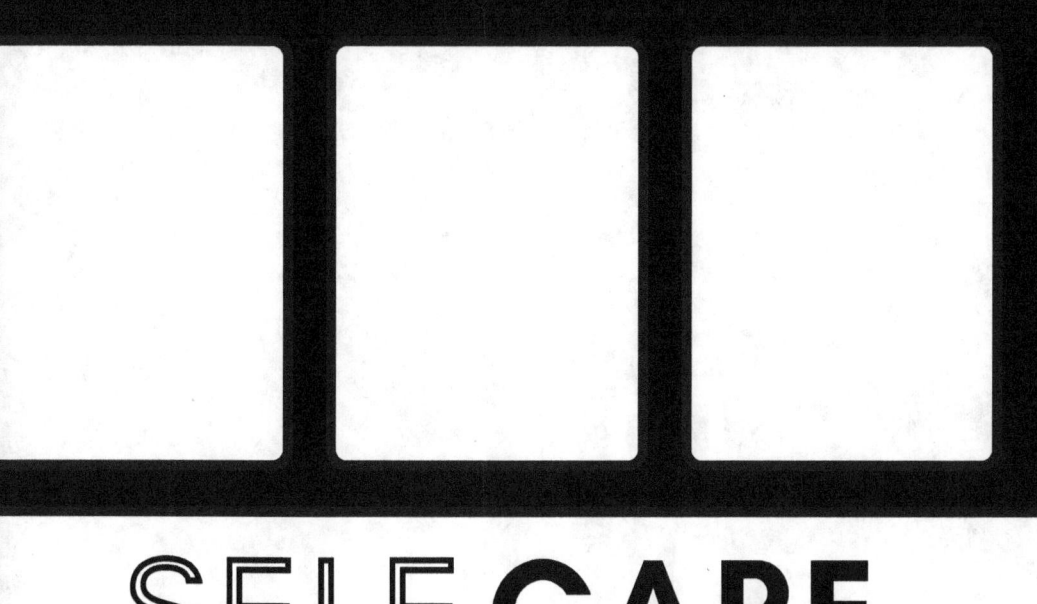

SELF CARE

In the boxes, describe and draw practical ways you can show yourself care

Rise

ABOVE

& BEYOND

Date: _____

SELF-CARE PLANNER

Date: _____ Month: _____ Year: _____

Today's Mood

☹ ☹ 😐 🙂 😃

Self-Care List

- .... ☐
- .... ☐
- .... ☐
- .... ☐
- .... ☐
- .... ☐
- .... ☐
- .... ☐

Things that made Me Happy Today

1. ....
2. ....
3. ....
4. ....
5. ....

Affirmation

....
....

Inspiration

....
....

Date:

LOVING ON MYSELF

Do I love myself enough to forgive others?

What are my boundaries in a friendship?

To Achieve all of These....

The Aspects For A Simple Love

Confidence

Pride

Will

Love

Happiness

Joy

Laughter

Share your thoughts on message!

Self-love

Date: ....

Month: ....

Year: ....

Things that made Me Happy Today:

....

....

....

....

....

Self-Care List

- ....
- ....
- ....
- ....

Priorities:

- _____
- _____
- _____
- _____
- _____

Dear Self:

....

....

....

Date:

STRONG IS THE NEW BEAUTIFUL

Date:

Self-love

Date: ....

Month: ....

Year: ....

Things that made Me Happy Today:

....

....

....

....

....

Self-Care List

- ....
- ....
- ....
- ....

Priorities:

- _____
- _____
- _____
- _____

Dear Self:

....

....

....

Date:

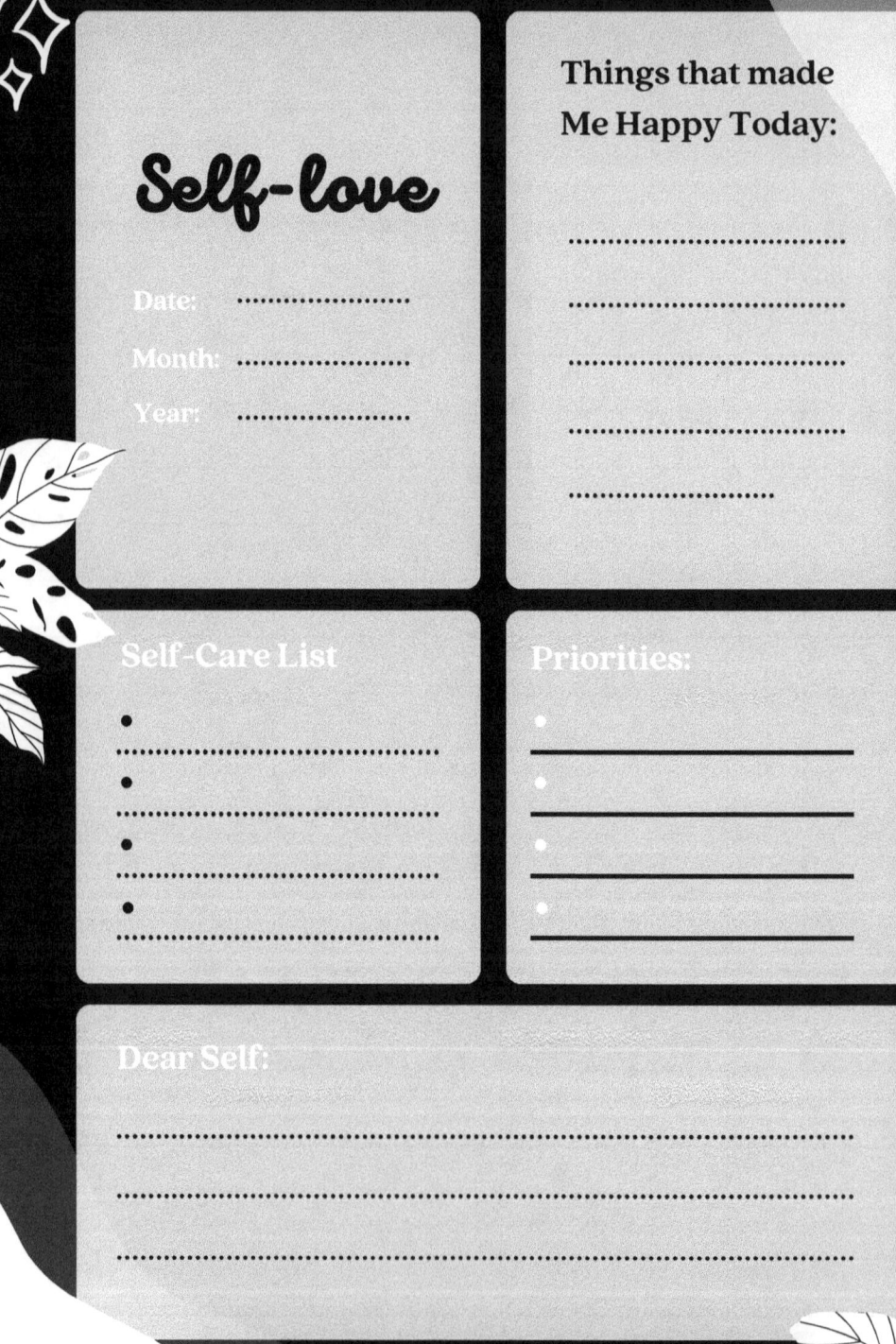

Self-love

Date: ....

Month: ....

Year: ....

Things that made Me Happy Today:

....

....

....

....

....

Self-Care List

- ....
- ....
- ....
- ....

Priorities:

- _____
- _____
- _____
- _____

Dear Self:

....

....

....

Date:

Self-love

Date: ....
Month: ....
Year: ....

Things that made Me Happy Today:

....
....
....
....
....

Self-Care List

- ....
- ....
- ....
- ....

Priorities:

- _____
- _____
- _____
- _____

Dear Self:

....
....
....

Date:

SELF-DISCOVERY

What is a very special but ordinary
memory you have that would not
really mean much to someone else
if you told them?

What's a random but vivid
memory you have that you'll never
forget, but doesn't really hold
much importance in your life?

What is something you're weirdly
good at without having had formal
training or much practice?

Is there a moment in your life that
you wish you could do over?
If yes, what is it and what would
you change?

When you were a kid, what did
you think you would do when you
grew up? How close were you?

Date:

Self-love

Date: ....

Month: ....

Year: ....

Things that made Me Happy Today:

....

....

....

....

....

Self-Care List

- ....
- ....
- ....
- ....

Priorities:

- _____
- _____
- _____
- _____

Dear Self:

....

....

....

Date:

Self-love

Date: ....

Month: ....

Year: ....

Things that made Me Happy Today:

....

....

....

....

....

Self-Care List

- ....
- ....
- ....
- ....

Priorities:

- _____
- _____
- _____
- _____

Dear Self:

....

....

....

Date:

SURVIVOR

Date:

Self-love

Date: ....

Month: ....

Year: ....

Things that made Me Happy Today:

....

....

....

....

....

Self-Care List

- ....
- ....
- ....
- ....

Priorities:

- _____
- _____
- _____
- _____

Dear Self:

....

....

....

Date:

Self-love

Date: ....

Month: ....

Year: ....

Things that made Me Happy Today:

....

....

....

....

....

Self-Care List

- ....
- ....
- ....
- ....

Priorities:

- _____
- _____
- _____
- _____

Dear Self:

....

....

....

Date:

A SELF-LOVE CHECKLIST

☐ Sleep at least seven hours a day

☐ Start your day with a protein or collagen

☐ Increase your intake of fresh fruits

☐ Drink at least 2 liters of water a day

☐ Relax with a good book

☐ Wear something that makes you feel good

☐ Spare time for your skin care

☐ Eat enough food to nourish your body

☐ Make sure to stretch your muscles

☐ Take a relaxing bath / shower

☐ Meditate for 15 minutes

☐ Go for a hike or a long walk in nature

☐ Be thankful for what you have got

_____

_____

Date:

WHAT ARE MY...

NOTE

_____
_____
_____
_____
_____
_____
_____
_____
_____
_____
_____
_____
_____
_____
_____
_____
_____
_____
_____
_____
_____
_____

 ☑ THOUGHTS

☑ FEELINGS

☑ BEHAVIOR

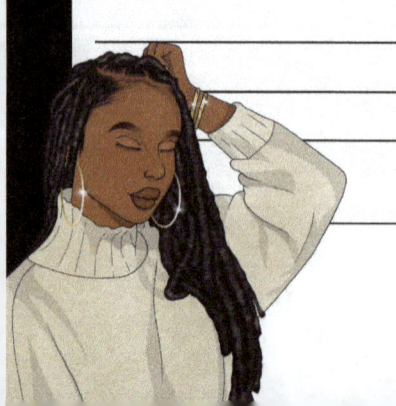

Date:

PUT YOURSELF FIRST

Date:

EVALUATE

TRACK YOUR GOALS TO MAKE IT MATTER!

Are my goals really what I want?

NOTE:

Can I rely on myself?

NOTE:

Do I believe I'm worthy of good things?

NOTE:

Do you love yourself enough to forgive yourself?

NOTE:

Do you love yourself enough to forgive others?

NOTE:

RESILIENCE

Date: _____

Date:

SELF-LOVE

STOP COMPARING YOURSELF TO OTHERS

01

ALLOW YOURSELF TO MAKE MISTAKES

02

DON'T WORRY ABOUT OTHERS' OPINIONS

03

Date:

DO YOU KNOW YOUR

LOVE LANGUAGE

Everyone's love language may not be the same. Have you found yours?

QUALITY TIME - Do Something By Yourself	**PHYSICAL TOUCH - Do Something For Your Body**
• Morning pages • Take a nap • Watch a movie you love • Go for a walk • Read a book you love • Fill your space with plants	• Set time to meditate • Exercise for 30 minutes • Yoga class • Take a bubble bath • Manicures/pedicures • Do a face mask
ACTS OF SERVICE - Do Something For Yourself	**RECEIVING GIFTS - Give Something to yourself**
• Cook a nice meal • Book travel ahead of time • Go to your favorite grocery • Clean your room • Do laundry • Wear your favorite outfit	• Treat yourself to a new book • Buy things for yourself • Knit yourself a scarf • Plan that vacation • Have a dance party • Order in dinner

Date:

WORDS OF AFFIRMATION

DO'S

👍 Give compliments often and make the detailed

👍 Send them a multiple texts to show you care

👍 Acknowledge them when they do something good

👍 Tell them why you appreciate them

👍 Find a variety of ways to incorporate words

DONT'S

👎 Don't give a fake word of affirmation

👎 Don't follow the above examples blindly

👎 Don't just affirm someone without giving reasons

👎 Don't say harsh words in a fit of anger

👎 Don't respond to them in short, scanty messages

Date:

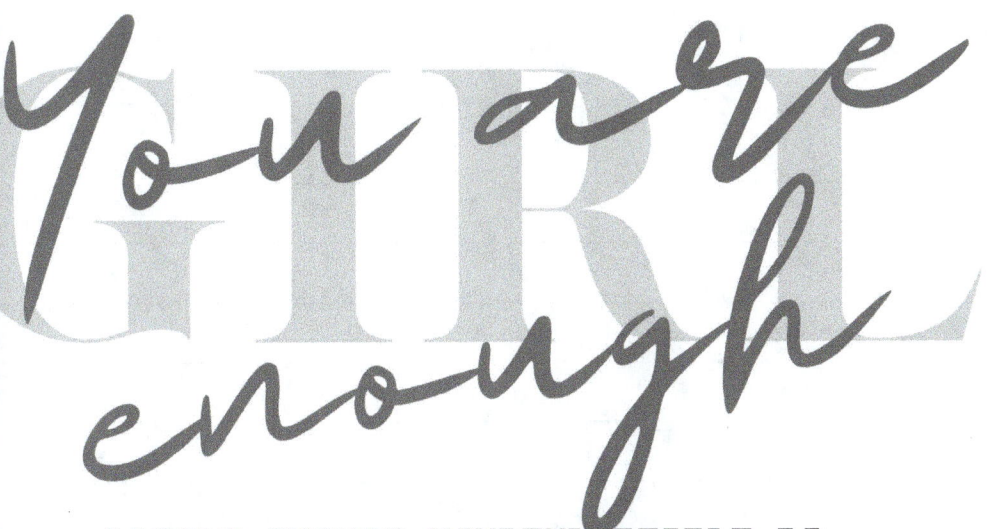

You are GIRL enough

LITTLE THINGS MINDFUL PEOPLE DO
DIFFERENTLY

- [x] *They Don't Multitask*
- [x] *They don't get hooked by their emotions*
- [x] *They get curious and ask questions*
- [x] *They embrace imperfection*
- [x] *They express their feelings*
- [x] *They know when to be quiet*
- [x] *They tap into their creativity*
- [x] *They focus on what they're doing*
- [x] *They Pause Before Reacting*
- [x] *They Watch Their Thoughts*
- [x] *They Engage In Self-Care*
- [x] *They Focus On Being A Good Listener*

Date:

FALL IN LOVE WITH
YOURSELF

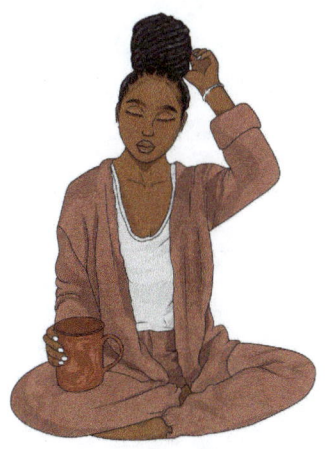

Self-love means knowing who you are as a whole and loving yourself anyway.

How do I express gratitude?

How often do I tell myself "I can't"?

Date:

My Week of Awesome

Priority Tasks

Upcoming Events

Don't Forget!

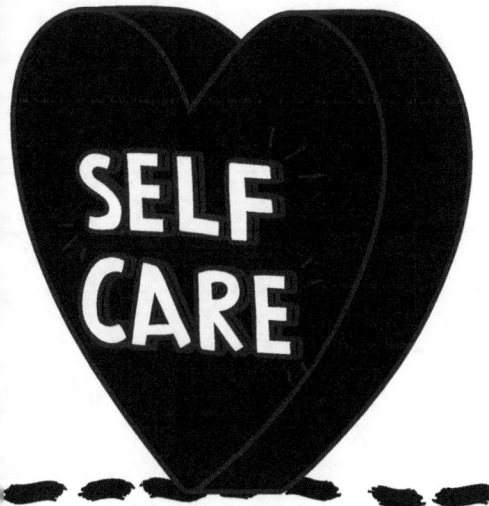

Date:

My Week of Awesome

Priority Tasks

Upcoming Events

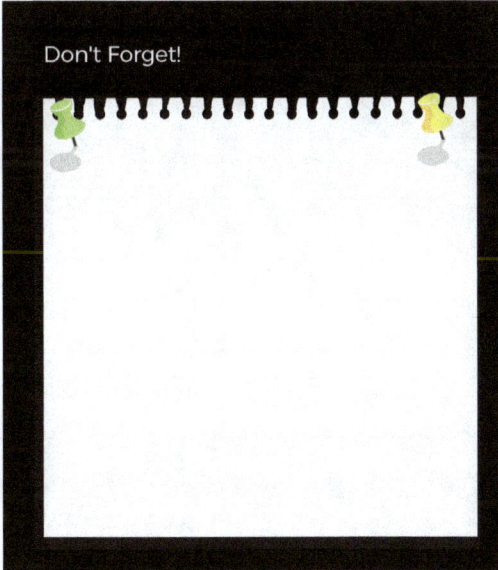
Don't Forget!

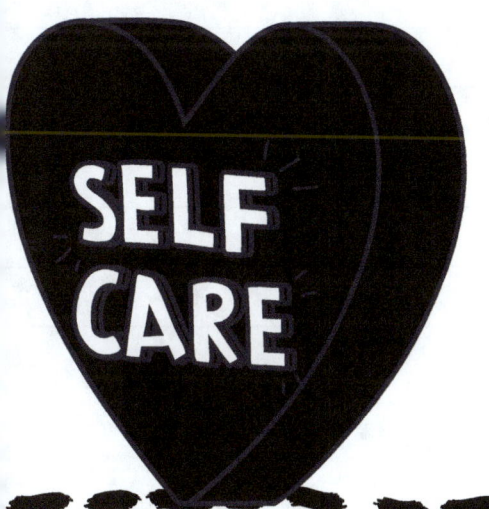

Date:

REFLECTION

ON MY JOURNEY TO SELF-LOVE

You're the
CEO of your life.
Be the leader
you need

Date:

BEING GRATEFUL FOR THE LITTLE BLESSINGS

I choose to make time
for peace and solitude.

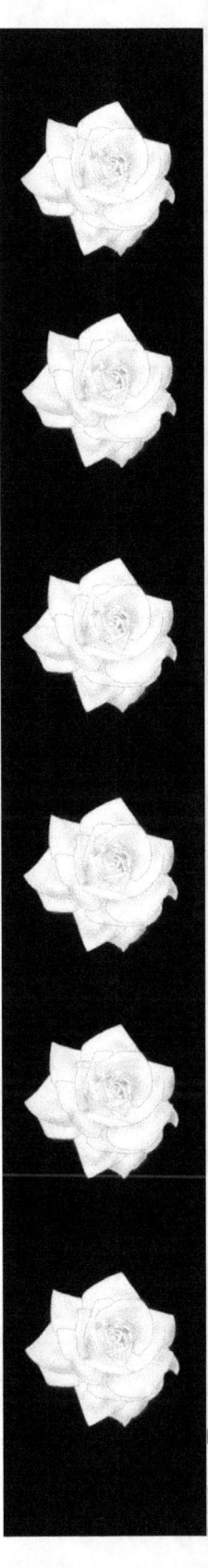

Date:

My Week of Awesome

Priority Tasks

Upcoming Events

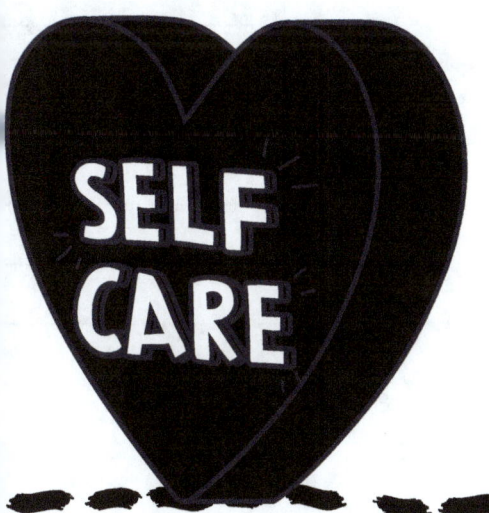

SELF CARE

Don't Forget!

Date:

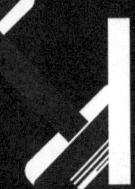

WORK IT!

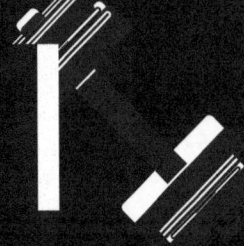

	ACTIVITY	TIME	REPS
DAY 1	• Stretching & warm-up • Tempo-run 3 miles • Chest and shoulders	20 min 1,.5 hrs 2 hrs.	5 times 1 round 20 reps
DAY 2	• Legs and cardio • Easy run 3 miles • Wall Tricep Pushes	1 hr 30 mins 1.5 hrs	30 reps 1 round 50 reps
DAY 3	• Stretching & warm-up • Tempo-run 3 miles • Chest and shoulders	20 min 1,.5 hrs 2 hrs.	5 times 1 round 20 reps
DAY 4	• Legs and cardio • Easy run 3 miles • Wall Tricep Pushes	1 hr 30 mins 1.5 hrs	30 reps 1 round 50 reps
DAY 5	• Stretching & warm-up • Tempo-run 3 miles • Chest and shoulders	20 min 1,.5 hrs 2 hrs.	5 times 1 round 20 reps

Date:

MY SELF—CARE
MASTER PLAN

It's time to put words and concepts into action. The changes that lead to extraordinary comes about born here. Please take whatever time you need to write down what you're willing to do to take better care of yourself in the moments. Please be concrete, specific and realistic.

PSYCHOLOGICAL SELF-CARE

_____

_____

_____

PHYSICAL SELF-CARE

_____

_____

_____

RELATIONSHIP/FAMILY SELF-CARE

_____

_____

_____

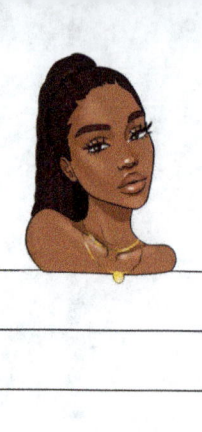

Date:

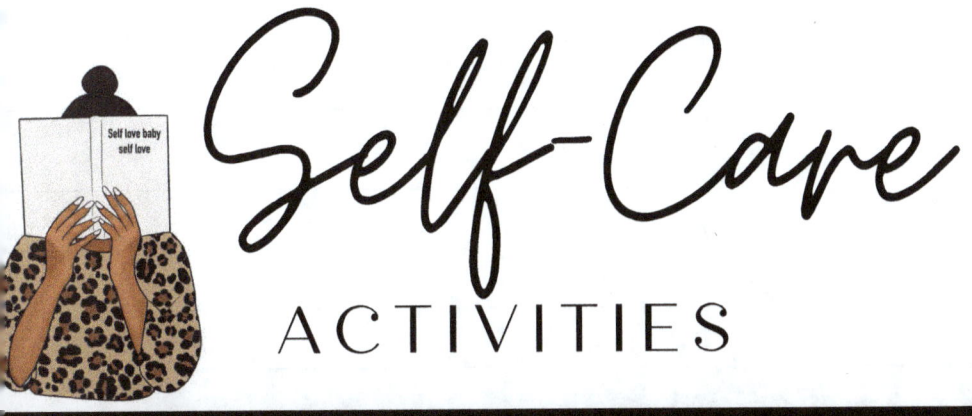

Self-Care
ACTIVITIES

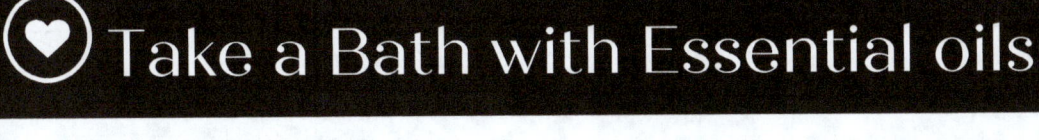

Take a Bath with Essential oils

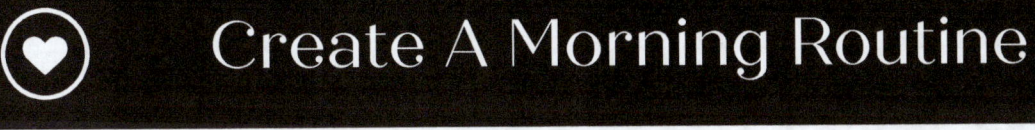

Create A Morning Routine

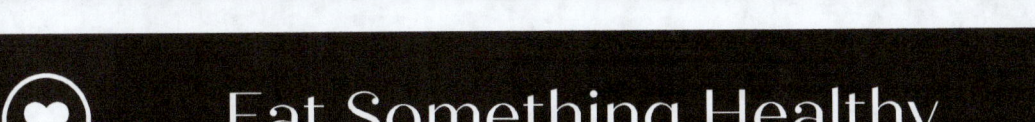

Eat Something Healthy

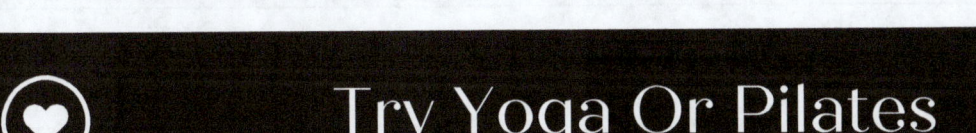

Try Yoga Or Pilates

Journal

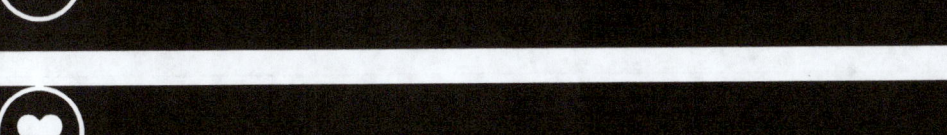

Aromatheraphy

Date:

SELF-LOVE POEM

You are not small.

You are not unworthy.

You are not insignificant.

The universe wove you from a constellation,

just so atom, every fibre in you comes from

a different star.

Together, you are bound by stardust , altogether

spectacularly created by the energy of the

universe itself.

And that, my darling,

is the poetry of physics,

the poetry of you.

—Nikita Gill

SENDING
VIRTUAL HUG

Thank you.

Every time you find humor in a difficult situation You Win
-Peanuts

loading..